My Appointment Notebook

Your Guide To Helping You Through Your Breast Cancer Journey

A Companion Book for *An Atypical Journey—Facing Breast Cancer Alone In The Middle East with God and My Tribe*

My Appointment Notebook

Your Guide To Helping You Through Your Breast Cancer Journey

A Companion Book for *An Atypical Journey—Facing Breast Cancer Alone In The Middle East with God and My Tribe*

V. Ronnie Laughlin

FRANKLIN GREEN
PUBLISHING
franklingreenpublishing.com

My Appointment Notebook
Your Guide To Helping You Through Your Breast Cancer Journey
A Companion Book for *An Atypical Journey— Facing Breast Cancer Alone In The Middle East with God and My Tribe*
By V. Ronnie Laughlin
Franklin Green Publishing
232 South St
Concord NH 03301
franklingreenpublishing.com

ISBN: 9781936487578

Editing: Heidi Jensen

Cover design: Heidi Jensen

Interior design: Kent Jensen | knail.com

Table Of Contents

Dedication

My Appointment Notebook is firstly dedicated to my Momma, Essie Laughlin, who always wrote down information and was very organized in her business. As a Beautician, she kept an appointment book for her customers, but she also wrote notes in her appointment book about events, people, and things in her life.

After my Momma's death in 2019, I found some of her appointment books. As I read through them, various types of notes were jotted down. My Momma had some notes about medications that she needed to take and the time she took them. It was just a little note like: 8:00 a.m. took pressure pill; the note would be followed by a check for noted it was done! She had days, times, and notes about when I called home from college and what we chatted about. She had notes about when things were due like. . . 'Get oil changed'. My Momma's appointment books were little windows into how she was organized and kept things together.

When I was diagnosed with Intraductal Carcinoma of my right breast while working and living alone in the Middle East, I knew that I would have to stay organized so that I could keep up with my medications, appointments, tests, etc. I started carrying a notebook with me to all my appointments. As time went on, I noticed a pattern of information that I was adding to the notebook with each visit. I found the notebook helpful in keeping me organized during my journey. Thanks, Momma, for instilling in me a need to be organized and document life as it happens around me.

My Appointment Notebook is also dedicated to my Mentor and Friend, Dr. Amelia Irby Hudson. Amelia was an academician who instilled in me the need to be accountable in all aspects of my life. When I thought about developing the parts of *My Appointment Notebook*, I thought about Amelia and all her copious notes that she took whenever she went to her appointments during her battles with breast, lung, and pancreatic cancers over the years. She was so organized and could always tell you what appointment was next and what her test results revealed. It was this sense of completeness and thoroughness that I channeled as I was molding and shaping the components of *My Appointment Notebook*. Amelia lost her cancer battle in 2021. I am forever grateful to her for her shining example of organizational skills and positive outlook during her journey.

My Appointment Notebook is also dedicated to my former Coach, Kay Yow. Coach Yow's very public breast cancer battle allowed the world to see how she managed her coaching, treatments, appointments and any setbacks that came along. I am most certain that Coach Yow had some kind of planner that she kept all of her medical information organized along with her practice and game schedules. Coach Yow was my example in how to keep moving forward in your cancer journey and know what is coming next. What a blessing it was to have seen Coach Yow smoothly manage her cancer journey in all aspects of her life.

My Appointment Notebook is also dedicated to anyone who has been on a cancer journey and has had to keep track of vital information. You too were in my thoughts as I thought about the composition and make-up of *My Appointment Notebook*. I wanted to make *My Appointment Notebook* logical and easy to follow. Having all my medical information in one spot, quelled my mind. I knew that I could jot down my questions for my doctors and make notes during my appointments. This behavior along with audio recordings of the appointments were helpful for me to gain understanding about my cancer and the procedures that I was going through. For me, there is nothing like written information that I can go to for reference.

Because there is a cancer protocol that you enter once you are diagnosed, the order of events, appointments, and procedures is similar in most cancer centers. I think you will find *My Appointment Notebook* easy to follow via a logical progression to augment your journey.

It is my sincere hope that *My Appointment Notebook* will bring you a sense of calm in knowing that all your medical information is in one place and that you feel confident in asking your prepared questions in a confident manner during your journey.

Here's to you for taking some good notes and information for keeping track of your journey!

Enjoy your *My Appointment Notebook*. Let me know how it works for you by sending an email tracking and documenting your journey to: info@ronnielaughlin.com

Happy tracking!!

We never realize what God is putting us through—we go through it more or less without understanding. Then suddenly, we come to a place of enlightenment and realize—*"God has strengthened me, and I did not even know it!"*

Introduction

How to Use My Appointment Notebook

Hello Dear Friend,

Thank you for purchasing *My Appointment Notebook*. This is the companion to my book *An Atypical Journey— Facing Breast Cancer Alone In The Middle East with God and My Tribe*. If you are starting your cancer journey, already in it, or are a caregiver, spouse, or Tribe member this is the perfect tool for your journey.

You have been tasked with having to undergo a series of rather complex medical treatments that will include many processes and procedures you may or may not be familiar with. Worry not, this book will be your guide to making sure you ask and get through all of the questions you have for your medical team, and keep track of all your appointments, treatments, exams, and meetings during your cancer journey.

This book will be a gem for you!

I came up with the idea, right after my diagnosis of breast cancer. Having had several friends who had undergone cancer treatments in the past, I was very familiar with the overall protocol and how overwhelming it can be.

There will be many twists and turns in your journey, but *My Appointment Notebook* will allow you to keep all your information in one handy, easy and accessible place for your use.

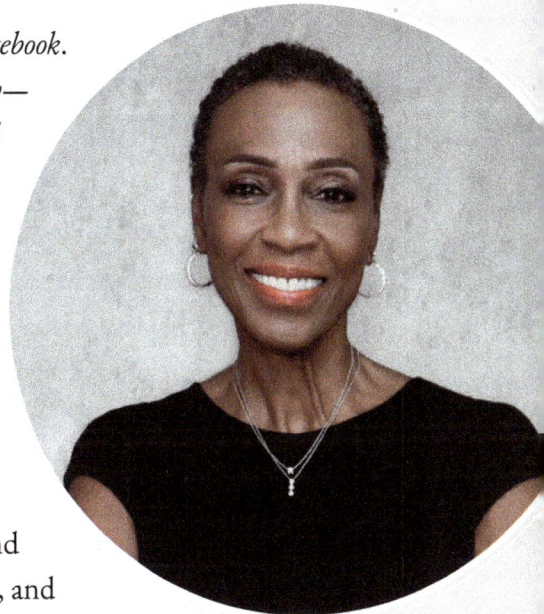

Also, do not forget to make voice memos during all your appointments. I found this very helpful and most of all comforting, as I could listen and take a few notes while in the appointment knowing that once I was back home, I could listen more closely and augment my notes with the information the doctors shared. Your memory and recall will not be as sharp as it was after going through chemo—trust me—chemo brain is real!

My Appointment Notebook is sectioned, and color coded and tabbed into the various types of appointments/disciplines you will encounter during your cancer journey. They are in the order that I had my appointments, but please feel free to use *My Appointment Notebook* in a way that best suits your needs. There are plenty of extra sheets in each section and at the end of the book.

SOME OF THE FEATURES OF *MY APPOINTMENT NOTEBOOK*

Words of Encouragement and Positive Thoughts

For each section on the adjacent page I have provided you with a few words of inspiration and encouragement to keep you focused and motivated. You will find a few of my insights, quotes or some of my words for a positive mindset to help you move through the journey. Feel free to add your own phrases or notes, and remember, this is YOUR Appointment Notebook that will be filled by and for you!

What You'll Find Ahead

Inside *My Appointment Notebook* are sheets for the following medical visits:

- General Medical
- OB-GYN
- Breast Surgeon
- Port Insertion
- Oncologist
- Cancer Counseling
- Radiologist
- Oncology/Chemo and Radiation

I have even given you a sample sheet completed so you can see how it can be filled in.

Also included are sections for your medical history, medications and allergies. There is a section for your contacts in a quick reference list format for your physicians, family members and friends.

Take a look at the sheets now to become familiar with their location in the book. I have also included a Table of Contents for easy accessibility.

Keeping Track

Each sheet is marked at the top for the type of visit, as well as color coded and tabbed. There is space for date, time in/out and for your vital signs. Keep track of your vital signs. It will provide vital information on your journey to ensure that you are not harboring any infections (high temps), losing or gaining weight, or other information that you and your doctor will need. I have included a space for you to track your oxygen saturation levels. These levels are vital for regulating your body to ensure that oxygen is getting to your organs (brain, heart, thyroid, kidneys) and to avoid any hypoxia (low level of oxygen). Hypoxia can lead to confusion, difficulty breathing, rapid heart rate, or restlessness. Your chemo will give you some of these symptoms, no point in complicating matters; something to be aware of for you and your caregiver.

On the sheets I have provided space for the purpose of your visit. It may be as simple as finding out test results of previous testing, or as complex as finding out your schedule for your chemo and the drugs that will be used. Try to keep in mind YOUR purpose for each specific visit.

Quiet Contemplation and Preparation

It will be very important for you to sit down in a quiet place a few days before your appointments, to think about the purpose of the specific appointment and questions that you will want to ask your doctor. My quiet times before my appointments allowed me to organize my thoughts and make sure I had covered everything that I needed and wanted to ask. Take the time to do this, and you will find that it's much less stressful when you don't have to think right there on the spot.

For your first OB-GYN visit, it may be to confirm suspicion of a mass/lesion like it was for me. I had lumps that needed to be palpated (touched) by a professional who knew what he/she was touching. That visit prompted the need for the ultrasound, biopsy, and mammogram and set the ball rolling for my journey.

I often got information from my Oncologist about what to ask my other doctors. Remember each doctor is disciplined in a specific matter but they do work together for your health care plan of treatment. So, write this information in you notebook too.

How To Be A Good Patient

Think of any questions you want to ask your doctor or staff. These will most likely be geared towards finding information about what procedures may be done, what to wear to the procedure, or any specific directives. This includes the medications to be given and their side effects. Remember, this is about YOU—so ask anything and everything you want to—but take my advice and use the sentence frames of: "Can you help me understand ..." or "I am wondering ...." This set up allows for an open and relaxed exchange between you and your medical staff. This makes it seem more like a conversation rather than a question-and-answer session. You want to establish a good rapport with your medical team, and this form of questioning is a great way of setting up that foundation.

I have included various prompts/questions depending on the visit. For example, for the Port-a-catheter insertion, I gave you more specific questions to be sure to ask the surgeon about the procedure, types of anesthesia, to show you the device, and pre-surgical instructions, etc.

Free Writing Space

Also included on your appointment sheets is space for notes for any consultations that are needed before or after the next appointment. Remember that you are now in a cancer protocol (official system of rules that explain the correct conduct and procedures to be followed in a medical situation).

Because you will be on a long protocol, I have included a space for you to jot down the names of the medical staff that you interact with. They may change or rotate in and out, but it is always nice to call the staff by name and engage in some conversational exchanges with them to make your visit pleasant and establish a good rapport.

You Will Be Tested Beyond Measure

When you have your appointment with your Breast Surgeon, you will move into the cancer protocol. Your plan of treatment has been established by the Tumor Board. It will start with the following visits:

Oncology—For your Oncology Appointments, it will be imperative you know the names of the drugs that you will receive and what their purpose is for your cancer battle. I have added space for listing the potential side effects from the drugs as well as space for the medications that you will have to take to quell your nausea and vomiting—keep track of this information, as it is extremely vital that you have little or no reaction to your chemo. Your Oncologist will tell you some of the common side effects. Do your research to find all the side effects so you are aware and alert of possible complications, if caught early it will help you progress on your journey.

Chemo—The Chemo Appointment Sheets will help you keep track of the drugs given during chemo, the times the IV was started and stopped and whether or not there were reactions. This information will be very beneficial in planning your schedule around the sessions. Knowing about how long your chemo sessions run will help you to manage your day. You will want to try to keep some kind of daily schedule for your newly created life with chemotherapy. There are eight appointment sheets. All thanks to God, I had four rounds of chemo. If you have to have more, there is space for you to document.

Remember, the first chemo treatment is long. They will give your chemo drugs via IV in a very slow drip to monitor any reaction you may have. Once there is no reaction noted, the drip will be increased. You will not be able to gauge your time in/out from your first round of chemo. Just know that your second round will be faster. Keep track of that second round of chemo. The times may vary slightly depending on the wait for the drugs. The chemo drugs are made as needed and there can be a wait—be patient and relax; believe in the system and the protocol.

Radiology—You will see that Radiology has a part I, II, IA and IIA. You will have to get a battery of tests from Radiology on two occasions. One as a baseline and the other as a follow-up after your treatment to determine effectiveness of the intervention. Your first visit to the Radiologist will probably be for an ultrasound and/or biopsy and mammogram (I). For example, I have included questions to ask the Radiologist about the ultrasound and mammogram such as the purpose of all the testing, what to expect, and any pre-procedural instructions that may be warranted. I have also included a few questions for the Radiologist for the MRI/CT visit (II). Of course, in the case of a suspected/confirmed malignancy, you will have all procedures for clarification and definition of the site of the lesion. I gave you space for responses to question about what to expect, and pre-procedures needed.

Your Radiology IA and IIA appointment sheets can be used for the repeat of the above procedures after your chemo or surgery is completed. You can make notes as needed on these sheets.

There Is An Easy Part; Believe It or Not

Radiation was easy in comparison to chemo for me. It is my prayer that it is easy for you as well. It is non-invasive and it goes very quickly. Embrace your radiation treatments as little rest periods from your chemo journey.

Radiation—Lastly, there is a Radiation appointment sheet that helps you track your radiation appointments, as they are typically daily (five days a week). I have divided the Radiation sheets into the initial appointment (I) and the subsequent appointments. Your initial appointment will be for measuring and aligning you for your radiation. Your appointments after that will be quick and easy, in and out with minimal questions. I have given you additional sheets to track your treatments.

Other Helpful Tips For Your Journey

My Appointment Notebook is my way of helping you keep things going smoothly along your journey. Use it, and enjoy it—I tried to include everything that I needed. Though your journey may be a bit different from mine; you may need more or less information. Nonetheless, use *My Appointment Notebook* accordingly and let me know how it works for you in your journey.

Be sure to keep it in a place where you will not forget to take it with you to your appointments. I had mine near my door so that when I picked up my purse, it was there to be seen and I always took it with me. I found *My Appointment Notebook* to be extremely beneficial, not to mention my medical team always expected me to refer to it with my questions during and after my appointments.

When I was receiving my chemo, I had a designated "chemo bag" that I carried with me to each session. I would carry all my necessities—my Kindle, as I got some reading done during my chemo drip. I also carried snacks of some kind—crackers or protein bars to nibble on. I had a pair of socks, along with a wrap or a shawl, as it was always cold during my sessions—it's nice to be prepared. Thankfully, the Oncology Department provided warm blankets and hot meals that I came to rely on. I kept a bottle of water with me wherever I went—hydration is so important. Pack what you need to be comfy for a few hours. Time will go slowly. You may want to pack your journal to jot a few thoughts down in, knitting or crocheting materials, a puzzle book—whatever you enjoy doing for a few hours. I know that this is "chemo" but God has allowed you this time to slow down and enjoy the simple things in life. Take this time to pray for those around you.

Since you have read my book, An Atypical Journey—you are now armed with good information about what to expect and you know some of the intricacies of the cancer protocol. With *My Appointment Notebook* in hand, you should feel confident in knowing that you will be able to track your journey with ease.

I am sending out my prayers and positivity your way for strength on your journey. Let me know how useful you found *My Appointment Notebook*. If you would like to make suggestions, leave me your comments and feedback at info@ronnielaughlin.com. I look forward to hearing from you.

Remember there is a method to the madness every step of the way. Unfortunately, there are not any short cuts in the cancer journey and protocol—be patient and believe in the process. It is tried and true!

Be well and keep moving forward in your journey—you've got this!

With Lots of Love Now and Beyond,

V. Ronnie Laughlin

www.ronnielaughlin.com

Appointment Sheets

Section One

Sample Appointment Sheet

When you're not feeling like
you have control over the
situation, stop, breathe and tell
yourself—I can do all things through
Christ who strengthens me;
Philippians 4:13—YOU'VE got this!

Medical Appointment <u>*Neurology*</u>

PHYSICIAN'S NAME: *Dr. Smith*
SPECIALTY AREA: *Neurology*
NURSE'S NAME: *Jana, Pricilla*

DATE: *6 May 2023*
TIME IN: *10:00*
TIME OUT: *10:45*
TOTAL: *45 minutes*

VITAL STATS
BP: *120/80* TEMP: *98.6* HT: *5ft 11* WT: *145* O_2 LEVEL: *90%*

PURPOSE/OBJECTIVE(S) OF APPOINTMENT: *To determine source of headaches and neck pain.*

QUESTIONS
1. *Could the headaches be related to stress—changed jobs recently?*

2. *Can neck pain be related to sleeping position—got new pillows that are not comfy?*

3. *I recently lowered my caffeine intake, could this be the source?*

NOTES: *Stress can be a source, but will need to r/o (rule out) tumor or lesion putting pressure on an area and causing the symptoms. May want to change pillows or adjust for better sleeping. Lowered caffeine intake can produce withdrawal symptoms—but not for long—worth the investigation to determine the cause.*

CONSULTATIONS NEEDED BEFORE NEXT APPOINTMENT:
Schedule MRI to investigate cause.

Section Two

Medical Appointment Sheets

Ronnie's
Words of Wisdom

My prayers are going out to you for
good health now and in the coming
days. Stay strong, positive and
moving forward in your journey.

Medical Appointment _____

DR.'S NAME: DATE:
                                               TIME IN:
NURSE'S NAME: TIME OUT:
                                               TOTAL:

VITAL STATS

BP: TEMP: HT: WT: O_2 LEVEL:

PURPOSE/OBJECTIVE(S) OF APPOINTMENT:

QUESTIONS FOR DOCTOR/MEDICAL STAFF

MEDICATIONS GIVEN:

NEXT APPOINTMENT:

NOTES:

CONSULTATIONS NEEDED BEFORE NEXT APPOINTMENT:

Ronnie's
Words of Wisdom

If you believe you can achieve good health; you can. Start slowly: eat healthy foods, drink plenty of water and keep moving—this really is all about you!

Medical Appointment _____

DR.'S NAME: DATE:

                                                     TIME IN:

NURSE'S NAME: TIME OUT:

                                                     TOTAL:

VITAL STATS

BP: TEMP: HT: WT: O_2 LEVEL:

PURPOSE/OBJECTIVE(S) OF APPOINTMENT:

QUESTIONS FOR DOCTOR/MEDICAL STAFF

MEDICATIONS GIVEN:

NEXT APPOINTMENT:

NOTES:

CONSULTATIONS NEEDED BEFORE NEXT APPOINTMENT:

Ronnie's Words of Wisdom

Remember, this is your health—
make it your priority to achieve a
healthy lifestyle.

Medical Appointment _____

DR.'S NAME:

NURSE'S NAME:

DATE:

TIME IN:

TIME OUT:

TOTAL:

VITAL STATS

BP: TEMP: HT: WT: O_2 LEVEL:

PURPOSE/OBJECTIVE(S) OF APPOINTMENT:

QUESTIONS FOR DOCTOR/MEDICAL STAFF

MEDICATIONS GIVEN:

NEXT APPOINTMENT:

NOTES:

CONSULTATIONS NEEDED BEFORE NEXT APPOINTMENT:

Ronnie's
Words of Wisdom

Listen carefully to your body—
it will speak to you every day—love it
and speak back, take care of it.
You will only get one.

Medical Appointment _____

DR.'S NAME: DATE:

TIME IN:

NURSE'S NAME: TIME OUT:

TOTAL:

VITAL STATS

BP: TEMP: HT: WT: O_2 LEVEL:

PURPOSE/OBJECTIVE(S) OF APPOINTMENT:

QUESTIONS FOR DOCTOR/MEDICAL STAFF

MEDICATIONS GIVEN:

NEXT APPOINTMENT:

NOTES:

CONSULTATIONS NEEDED BEFORE NEXT APPOINTMENT:

Section Three

OB-GYN
Appointment Sheets

Ronnie's Words of Wisdom

Be strong and confident. You have made your annual breast and pelvic exams appointment! Congratulations—Well done!

OB-GYN Appointment

DR.'S NAME:

NURSE'S NAME:

DATE:

TIME IN:

TIME OUT:

TOTAL:

VITAL STATS

BP: TEMP: HT: WT: O_2 LEVEL:

PURPOSE/OBJECTIVE(S) OF APPOINTMENT:

PALPITATION OF BREASTS—

LEFT: RIGHT:

MAMMOGRAM:

ULTRASOUND:

PELVIC EXAM:

OTHER ADDITIONAL TESTS:

19

OB-GYN Appointment

QUESTIONS FOR DOCTOR/MEDICAL STAFF:

NOTES:

OB-GYN Appointment

NOTES:

CONSULTATIONS NEEDED BEFORE NEXT APPOINTMENT:

Ronnie's Words of Wisdom

Follow-up if needed in a
timely manner with any tests or
consultations—your goal:
A happy and healthy life!

OB-GYN Appointment

DR.'S NAME: DATE:

TIME IN:

NURSE'S NAME: TIME OUT:

TOTAL:

VITAL STATS

BP: TEMP: HT: WT: O$_2$ LEVEL:

PURPOSE/OBJECTIVE(S) OF APPOINTMENT:

PALPITATION OF BREASTS

LEFT: RIGHT:

MAMMOGRAM:

ULTRASOUND:

PELVIC EXAM:

OTHER ADDITIONAL TESTS:

OB-GYN Appointment

QUESTIONS FOR DOCTOR/MEDICAL STAFF:

NOTES:

OB-GYN Appointment

NOTES:

CONSULTATIONS NEEDED BEFORE NEXT APPOINTMENT:

Section Four

Breast Surgeon
Appointment Sheets

Ronnie's
Words of Wisdom

Your level of rapport and comfort with your medical team will be an asset in your overall recovery. Try to gain a level of trust and confidence with the medical team. This will help in your overall healing. Your patience will be tested; stay focused and keep moving forward!

Breast Surgeon Appointment

DR.'S NAME:

NURSE'S NAME:

DATE:

TIME IN:

TIME OUT:

TOTAL:

VITAL STATS

BP: TEMP: HT: WT: O_2 LEVEL:

PURPOSE/OBJECTIVE(S) OF APPOINTMENT:

QUESTIONS FOR SURGEON

TYPE OF CANCER—IF KNOWN:

SIZE OF MASS/TUMOR:

LOCATION:

INFORMATION TO RECEIVE: *Ask to review the ultrasound, mammogram results with the surgeon if done.*

Breast Surgeon Appointment

ADDITIONAL TESTS FROM THE BIOPSY

IHC (IMMUNOHISTOCHEMISTRY):

BRCA 1:

BRCA 2:

HER2:

OTHER ADDITIONAL TESTS

MRI:

CT SCAN:

PLAN FOR REMOVAL:

MAPPED OUT PLAN OF CARE:

WHAT IS THE NEXT STEP:

WHAT ARE ALL TESTS THAT NEED TO BE DONE:

Breast Surgeon Appointment

GAIN UNDERSTANDING OF THE TUMOR BOARD:

NEXT STEPS:

NOTES:

NEXT APPOINTMENT:

CONSULTATIONS NEEDED BEFORE NEXT APPOINTMENT:

Ronnie's
Words of Wisdom

Share your family history with your
Breast Surgeon. It is imperative
that he/she know about your breast
health and that of your family.

Breast Surgeon Appointment

DR.'S NAME:

DATE:

TIME IN:

NURSE'S NAME:

TIME OUT:

TOTAL:

VITAL STATS

BP:　　　　　TEMP:　　　　　HT:　　　　　WT:　　　　　O_2 LEVEL:

PURPOSE/OBJECTIVE(S) OF APPOINTMENT:

QUESTIONS FOR SURGEON

TYPE OF CANCER—IF KNOWN:

SIZE OF MASS/TUMOR:

LOCATION:

INFORMATION TO RECEIVE: *Ask to review the ultrasound, mammogram results with the surgeon if done.*

Breast Surgeon Appointment

ADDITIONAL TESTS FROM THE BIOPSY

IHC (IMMUNOHISTOCHEMISTRY):

BRCA 1:

BRCA 2:

HER2:

OTHER ADDITIONAL TESTS

MRI:

CT SCAN:

PLAN FOR REMOVAL:

MAPPED OUT PLAN OF CARE:

WHAT IS THE NEXT STEP:

WHAT ARE ALL TESTS THAT NEED TO BE DONE:

Breast Surgeon Appointment

GAIN UNDERSTANDING OF THE TUMOR BOARD:

NEXT STEPS:

NOTES:

NEXT APPOINTMENT:

CONSULTATIONS NEEDED BEFORE NEXT APPOINTMENT:

Breast Surgeon Appointment

DR.'S NAME:

DATE:

TIME IN:

NURSE'S NAME:

TIME OUT:

TOTAL:

VITAL STATS

BP: TEMP: HT: WT: O_2 LEVEL:

PURPOSE/OBJECTIVE(S) OF APPOINTMENT:

QUESTIONS FOR SURGEON

RESULTS OF SURGERY:

SENTINEL NODES POSITIVE OR NEGATIVE:

OTHER ADDITIONAL TESTS:

Breast Surgeon Appointment

MAPPED OUT PLAN OF CARE:

WHAT IS THE NEXT STEP:

WHAT ARE ALL THE TESTS THAT NEED TO BE DONE:

NEXT STEPS:

Breast Surgeon Appointment

NOTES:

NEXT APPOINTMENT DATE:

CONSULTATIONS NEEDED BEFORE NEXT APPOINTMENT:

Ronnie's
Words of Wisdom

Remember—try to use
your Appointment Notebook
consistently. A few days before
your appointment, take a few
moments in a quiet place and
gather your thoughts about the
appointment. Jot down any
questions that may arise.

Breast Surgeon Appointment

DR.'S NAME:

NURSE'S NAME:

DATE:

TIME IN:

TIME OUT:

TOTAL:

VITAL STATS

BP: TEMP: HT: WT: O_2 LEVEL:

PURPOSE/OBJECTIVE(S) OF APPOINTMENT:

QUESTIONS FOR SURGEON

RESULTS OF ULTRASOUND:

MAMMOGRAM AFTER SURGERY:

MRI AFTER SURGERY:

Breast Surgeon Appointment

CT AFTER SURGERY:

SENTINEL NODES:

LYMPH NODES:

NEXT STEPS:

Breast Surgeon Appointment

NOTES:

NEXT APPOINTMENT DATE:

CONSULTATIONS NEEDED BEFORE NEXT APPOINTMENT:

Section Five

Radiology I
Appointment Sheet

Ultrasound and Mammogram

Ronnie's
Words of Wisdom

Congrats on getting your
breast exam! Well done. Be sure to
ask questions. If God brings you to
it, He will surely bring you through it!
Stay positive! Start loving the idea
of taking care of you!

Radiology I Appointment – Ultrasound and Mammogram

RADIOLOGIST'S NAME: DATE:

                                                 TIME IN:

RADIOLOGY TECHNICIAN'S NAME: TIME OUT:

                                                 TOTAL:

VITAL STATS

BP: TEMP: HT: WT: O_2 LEVEL:

PURPOSE/OBJECTIVE(S) OF APPOINTMENT: *(Mention family history if applicable)*

_____

_____

_____

_____

QUESTIONS FOR RADIOLOGIST

PURPOSE?

_____

_____

WHAT TO EXPECT?

_____

_____

LENGTH OF TIME OF EACH PROCEDURE?

_____

_____

PURPOSE OF ULTRASOUND?

_____

_____

Radiology I Appointment – Ultrasound and Mammogram

BIOPSY NEEDED?

RESULTS FROM BIOPSY WILL BE BACK WHEN?

PURPOSE OF MAMMOGRAM?

WHAT TO EXPECT:

LENGTH OF TIME OF EACH PROCEDURE:

PRE-PROCEDURE INSTRUCTIONS:

WHAT TO WEAR:

EATING BEFORE PROCEDURE:

Radiology I Appointment – Ultrasound and Mammogram

NOTES:

CONSULTATIONS NEEDED BEFORE NEXT APPOINTMENT:

Section Six

Radiology IA Appointment Sheet

MRI/CT

Ronnie's
Words of Wisdom

The MRI and CT scan
can be a bit daunting. Relax and
breathe. Conjure up a pleasant and
funny thought or two that you can
focus on in all the chaos. After all,
the procedures only last a short
while! You have the stamina for it!
I believe in you!

Radiology IA Appointment – MRI/CT

RADIOLOGIST'S NAME: DATE:

                                        TIME IN:

RADIOLOGY TECHNICIAN'S NAME: TIME OUT:

                                          TOTAL:

VITAL STATS

BP: TEMP: HT: WT: O_2 LEVEL:

PURPOSE/OBJECTIVE(S) OF APPOINTMENT:

QUESTIONS FOR RADIOLOGIST

ARE THE PROCEDURES WITH OR WITHOUT CONTRAST? *(FYI—get rid of the contrast with lots of water afterwards.)*

WHAT TO EXPECT—CT SCAN: *(Any instructions for dress/eating prior to?)*

Radiology IA Appointment – MRI/CT

WHAT TO EXPECT—MRI: *(Any instructions for dress/eating prior to?)*

NOTES:

Radiology IA Appointment – MRI/CT

NOTES:

CONSULTATIONS NEEDED BEFORE NEXT APPOINTMENT:

Section Seven

Oncology
Appointment Sheets

Ronnie's Words of Wisdom

Remember—try not to stress about the process. Gather your spiritual, mental, physical, emotional and psychological strength—this is not a sprint! It is YOUR marathon for life, embrace it and pace yourself.

Oncology Appointment

ONCOLOGIST'S NAME:

DATE:

TIME IN:

NURSE'S NAME:

TIME OUT:

TOTAL:

VITAL STATS

BP: TEMP: HT: WT: O_2 LEVEL:

PURPOSE/OBJECTIVE(S) OF APPOINTMENT:

QUESTIONS FOR ONCOLOGIST

SURVIVAL RATE WITHOUT CHEMO (IF YOU WANT TO KNOW):

SURVIVAL RATE WITH CHEMO (IF YOU WANT TO KNOW):

RESULTS FROM THE TUMOR BOARD:

NUMBER OF ROUNDS:

Oncology Appointment

TYPE OF CHEMO:

NEOADJUVANT VS. ADJUVANT:

NAMES OF CHEMO DRUGS—

DRUG:

PURPOSE:

SIDE EFFECTS:

DRUG:

PURPOSE:

SIDE EFFECTS:

DRUG:

PURPOSE:

SIDE EFFECTS:

INJECTIONS TO BE GIVEN:

Oncology Appointment

MEDICATIONS TO BE TAKEN PRIOR TO CHEMO:

PURPOSE:

BLOOD WORK NEEDED BEFORE CHEMO:

NOTES:

CANCER COUNSELING:

NEXT APPOINTMENT:

CONSULTATIONS NEEDED BEFORE NEXT APPOINTMENT:

Oncology Appointment

ONCOLOGIST'S NAME: DATE:

                                            TIME IN:

NURSE'S NAME: TIME OUT:

                                            TOTAL:

VITAL STATS

BP: TEMP: HT: WT: O_2 LEVEL:

PURPOSE/OBJECTIVE(S) OF APPOINTMENT:

QUESTIONS FOR ONCOLOGIST

RESULTS FROM THE TUMOR BOARD:

NUMBER OF ROUNDS:

Oncology Appointment

TYPE OF CHEMO:

NEOADJUVANT VS. ADJUVANT:

NAMES OF CHEMO DRUGS—

DRUG:

PURPOSE:

SIDE EFFECTS:

DRUG:

PURPOSE:

SIDE EFFECTS:

DRUG:

PURPOSE:

SIDE EFFECTS:

INJECTIONS TO BE GIVEN:

Oncology Appointment

MEDICATIONS TO BE TAKEN PRIOR TO CHEMO:

PURPOSE:

BLOOD WORK NEEDED BEFORE CHEMO:

NOTES:

CANCER COUNSELING:

NEXT APPOINTMENT:

CONSULTATIONS NEEDED BEFORE NEXT APPOINTMENT:

Ronnie's Words of Wisdom

Remember to keep track of the vocabulary that you will be exposed to—understand it so that you can share with others in a knowledgeable way.

Oncology Appointment

ONCOLOGIST'S NAME: DATE:

TIME IN:

NURSE'S NAME: TIME OUT:

TOTAL:

VITAL STATS

BP: TEMP: HT: WT: O_2 LEVEL:

PURPOSE/OBJECTIVE(S) OF APPOINTMENT:

QUESTIONS FOR ONCOLOGIST

RESULTS FROM THE TUMOR BOARD:

NUMBER OF ROUNDS:

Oncology Appointment

TYPE OF CHEMO:

NEOADJUVANT VS. ADJUVANT:

NAMES OF CHEMO DRUGS—

DRUG:

PURPOSE:

SIDE EFFECTS:

DRUG:

PURPOSE:

SIDE EFFECTS:

DRUG:

PURPOSE:

SIDE EFFECTS:

INJECTIONS TO BE GIVEN:

Oncology Appointment

MEDICATIONS TO BE TAKEN PRIOR TO CHEMO:

PURPOSE:

BLOOD WORK NEEDED BEFORE CHEMO:

NOTES:

CANCER COUNSELING:

NEXT APPOINTMENT:

CONSULTATIONS NEEDED BEFORE NEXT APPOINTMENT:

Ronnie's Words of Wisdom

Always do a self-check-in
to make sure all your bases are
covered: How are you feeling?
Anything you need to share with
the Oncologist? Are you still having
moments where positive thoughts
are being made? Your mental
strength is just as important
as your physical strength.

Oncology Appointment

ONCOLOGIST'S NAME: DATE:

                                            TIME IN:

NURSE'S NAME: TIME OUT:

                                            TOTAL:

VITAL STATS

BP: TEMP: HT: WT: O_2 LEVEL:

PURPOSE/OBJECTIVE(S) OF APPOINTMENT:

QUESTIONS FOR ONCOLOGIST

RESULTS FROM THE TUMOR BOARD:

NUMBER OF ROUNDS:

Oncology Appointment

TYPE OF CHEMO:

NEOADJUVANT VS. ADJUVANT:

NAMES OF CHEMO DRUGS—

DRUG:

 PURPOSE:

 SIDE EFFECTS:

DRUG:

 PURPOSE:

 SIDE EFFECTS:

DRUG:

 PURPOSE:

 SIDE EFFECTS:

INJECTIONS TO BE GIVEN:

Oncology Appointment

MEDICATIONS TO BE TAKEN PRIOR TO CHEMO:

PURPOSE:

BLOOD WORK NEEDED BEFORE CHEMO:

NOTES:

CANCER COUNSELING:

NEXT APPOINTMENT:

CONSULTATIONS NEEDED BEFORE NEXT APPOINTMENT:

Section Eight

Cancer Counseling Appointment Sheet

Ronnie's Words of Wisdom

Getting information about what is going to be the sequence of events in your journey is vital. Embrace the information, understand it so that you are emboldened with knowledge about your health—take comfort in knowing that you know about your health plan.

Cancer Counseling Appointment

COUNSELOR'S NAME:

MEDICAL STAFF NAMES:

DATE:

TIME IN:

TIME OUT:

TOTAL:

VITAL STATS

BP: TEMP: HT: WT: O_2 LEVEL:

PURPOSE/OBJECTIVE(S) OF APPOINTMENT: *To learn and gather information about managing your cancer treatment; your mental and physical health during the cancer journey.*

QUESTIONS TO ASK

TIMELINES FOR CHEMO:

DRUGS TO BE USED:

EFFECTS OF DRUGS:

PRECAUTIONS FOR EATING:

FOOD GROUPS:

ORAL CARE:

EXERCISE:

Cancer Counseling Appointment

REST NEEDED DURING CHEMO, RADIATION, SURGERY:

HOW TO DEAL WITH CONSTIPATION: *water consumption, high fiber diet, exercise*

ADDITIONAL DRUGS TO BE TAKEN FOR NAUSEA/VOMITING:

WHAT ARE THE WARNING SIGNS TO WATCH FOR: *high fever, rashes, abdominal pain*

SUPPORT GROUPS:

NOTES:

Cancer Counseling Appointment

NOTES:

Section Nine

Port-a-Catheter Insertion Appointment Sheet

The port-a-catheter will make your chemo treatments go smoothly. Again, be patient with getting your head around the fact you have a small device in your chest. The port makes your life during chemo easier—you need something easy now—go with it!

Port-a-Catheter Insertion Appointment

SURGEON'S NAME:

DATE:

TIME IN:

NURSE'S NAME:

TIME OUT:

TOTAL:

VITAL STATS

BP: TEMP: HT: WT: O_2 LEVEL:

PURPOSE/OBJECTIVE(S) OF APPOINTMENT:

QUESTIONS FOR SURGEON

PROCEDURE FOR THE INSERTION:

TWILIGHT OR GENERAL ANESTHESIA:

RECOVERY TIME:

AFTER CARE:

Port-a-Catheter Insertion Appointment

INFORMATION TO RECEIVE:

EXPLANATION OF PROCEDURE:

SEE THE PORT-A-CATHETER:

DETERMINE THE SIDE OF THE INSERTION:

WHAT ARE THE PRECAUTIONS:

PRE-SURGICAL INSTRUCTIONS—
WHAT TO WEAR:

EATING PRIOR TO SURGERY:

RECOVERY TIME:

Port-a-Catheter Insertion Appointment

NOTES:

INSERTION APPOINTMENT DATE:

CONSULTATIONS NEEDED BEFORE NEXT APPOINTMENT:

Section Ten

Chemotherapy Appointment Sheets

We never realize what God is
putting us through—we go through it
more or less without understanding.
Then suddenly, we come to a place
of enlightenment and realize—
"God has strengthened me, and
I did not even know it!" Use the
time during your chemo sessions
to understand that you will be
stronger after this ordeal.

Chemotherapy Appointment – Round # ___

ONCOLOGIST'S NAME:

DATE:

TIME IN:

MEDICAL STAFF NAME:

TIME OUT:

TOTAL:

VITAL STATS

BP: TEMP: HT: WT: O_2 LEVEL:

PURPOSE/OBJECTIVE(S) OF APPOINTMENT:

QUESTIONS FOR MEDICAL STAFF

CHEMO DRUGS GIVEN AND TIME

DRUG: TIME START: TIME END:

  REACTION(S):

DRUG: TIME START: TIME END:

  REACTION(S):

DRUG: TIME START: TIME END:

  REACTION(S):

Chemotherapy Appointment – Round # ___

INJECTIONS GIVEN:

RIGHT BODY PART:

LEFT BODY PART:

ADDITIONAL DRUGS TO BE TAKEN FOR NAUSEA/VOMITING:

WHAT ARE THE WARNING SIGNS TO WATCH FOR: *high fever, rashes, abdominal pain*

NOTES:

Chemotherapy Appointment – Round # ___

NOTES:

Chemotherapy Appointment – Round # ____

ONCOLOGIST'S NAME:

MEDICAL STAFF NAME:

DATE:

TIME IN:

TIME OUT:

TOTAL:

VITAL STATS

BP: TEMP: HT: WT: O_2 LEVEL:

PURPOSE/OBJECTIVE(S) OF APPOINTMENT:

QUESTIONS FOR MEDICAL STAFF

CHEMO DRUGS GIVEN AND TIME

DRUG: TIME START: TIME END:

  REACTION(S):

DRUG: TIME START: TIME END:

  REACTION(S):

DRUG: TIME START: TIME END:

  REACTION(S):

Chemotherapy Appointment – Round # ___

INJECTIONS GIVEN:

RIGHT BODY PART:

LEFT BODY PART:

ADDITIONAL DRUGS TO BE TAKEN FOR NAUSEA/VOMITING:

WHAT ARE THE WARNING SIGNS TO WATCH FOR: *high fever, rashes, abdominal pain*

NOTES:

Chemotherapy Appointment – Round # ___

NOTES:

Ronnie's
Words of Wisdom

Give yourself credit for coming
this far! You are a champion!

Chemotherapy Appointment – Round # ___

ONCOLOGIST'S NAME:

DATE:

TIME IN:

MEDICAL STAFF NAME:

TIME OUT:

TOTAL:

VITAL STATS

BP: TEMP: HT: WT: O_2 LEVEL:

PURPOSE/OBJECTIVE(S) OF APPOINTMENT:

QUESTIONS FOR MEDICAL STAFF

CHEMO DRUGS GIVEN AND TIME

DRUG: TIME START: TIME END:

REACTION(S):

DRUG: TIME START: TIME END:

REACTION(S):

DRUG: TIME START: TIME END:

REACTION(S):

Chemotherapy Appointment – Round # ___

INJECTIONS GIVEN:

RIGHT BODY PART:

LEFT BODY PART:

ADDITIONAL DRUGS TO BE TAKEN FOR NAUSEA/VOMITING:

WHAT ARE THE WARNING SIGNS TO WATCH FOR: *high fever, rashes, abdominal pain*

NOTES:

Chemotherapy Appointment – Round # ___

NOTES:

Ronnie's Words of Wisdom

When "The Beast" appears, you will know!—ask your Oncologist about methylphenidate to combat your cancer related fatigue (CRF).

Chemotherapy Appointment – Round # ___

ONCOLOGIST'S NAME: DATE:

                                             TIME IN:

MEDICAL STAFF NAME: TIME OUT:

                                             TOTAL:

VITAL STATS

BP: TEMP: HT: WT: O_2 LEVEL:

PURPOSE/OBJECTIVE(S) OF APPOINTMENT:

QUESTIONS FOR MEDICAL STAFF

CHEMO DRUGS GIVEN AND TIME

DRUG: TIME START: TIME END:

  REACTION(S):

DRUG: TIME START: TIME END:

  REACTION(S):

DRUG: TIME START: TIME END:

  REACTION(S):

Chemotherapy Appointment – Round # ___

INJECTIONS GIVEN:

RIGHT BODY PART:

LEFT BODY PART:

ADDITIONAL DRUGS TO BE TAKEN FOR NAUSEA/VOMITING:

WHAT ARE THE WARNING SIGNS TO WATCH FOR: *high fever, rashes, abdominal pain*

NOTES:

Chemotherapy Appointment – Round # ___

NOTES:

Ronnie's Words of Wisdom

Having hair loss? You are
on your way to becoming the
new YOU! Embrace the new YOU!
Love the new YOU!

Chemotherapy Appointment – Round # ___

ONCOLOGIST'S NAME:

MEDICAL STAFF NAME:

DATE:

TIME IN:

TIME OUT:

TOTAL:

VITAL STATS

BP: TEMP: HT: WT: O_2 LEVEL:

PURPOSE/OBJECTIVE(S) OF APPOINTMENT:

QUESTIONS FOR MEDICAL STAFF

CHEMO DRUGS GIVEN AND TIME

DRUG: TIME START: TIME END:

 REACTION(S):

DRUG: TIME START: TIME END:

 REACTION(S):

DRUG: TIME START: TIME END:

 REACTION(S):

Chemotherapy Appointment – Round # ___

INJECTIONS GIVEN:

RIGHT BODY PART:

LEFT BODY PART:

ADDITIONAL DRUGS TO BE TAKEN FOR NAUSEA/VOMITING:

WHAT ARE THE WARNING SIGNS TO WATCH FOR: *high fever, rashes, abdominal pain*

NOTES:

Chemotherapy Appointment – Round #___

NOTES:

Ronnie's
Words of Wisdom

Tired? Take a nap—get refreshed.
Never feel guilty about resting and
taking care and taking
care of yourself!

Chemotherapy Appointment – Round # ___

ONCOLOGIST'S NAME:

DATE:

TIME IN:

MEDICAL STAFF NAME:

TIME OUT:

TOTAL:

VITAL STATS

BP: TEMP: HT: WT: O_2 LEVEL:

PURPOSE/OBJECTIVE(S) OF APPOINTMENT:

QUESTIONS FOR MEDICAL STAFF

CHEMO DRUGS GIVEN AND TIME

DRUG: TIME START: TIME END:

REACTION(S):

DRUG: TIME START: TIME END:

REACTION(S):

DRUG: TIME START: TIME END:

REACTION(S):

Chemotherapy Appointment – Round # ___

INJECTIONS GIVEN:

RIGHT BODY PART:

LEFT BODY PART:

ADDITIONAL DRUGS TO BE TAKEN FOR NAUSEA/VOMITING:

WHAT ARE THE WARNING SIGNS TO WATCH FOR: *high fever, rashes, abdominal pain*

NOTES:

Chemotherapy Appointment – Round # __

NOTES:

Ronnie's
Words of Wisdom

Moving forward is first in
your mind. Each day you get
through you are moving forward—
feel good about that!

Chemotherapy Appointment – Round # ___

ONCOLOGIST'S NAME: DATE:

                                                            TIME IN:

MEDICAL STAFF NAME: TIME OUT:

                                                            TOTAL:

VITAL STATS

BP: TEMP: HT: WT: O_2 LEVEL:

PURPOSE/OBJECTIVE(S) OF APPOINTMENT:

QUESTIONS FOR MEDICAL STAFF

CHEMO DRUGS GIVEN AND TIME

DRUG: TIME START: TIME END:

  REACTION(S):

DRUG: TIME START: TIME END:

  REACTION(S):

DRUG: TIME START: TIME END:

  REACTION(S):

Chemotherapy Appointment – Round # ___

INJECTIONS GIVEN:

RIGHT BODY PART:

LEFT BODY PART:

ADDITIONAL DRUGS TO BE TAKEN FOR NAUSEA/VOMITING:

WHAT ARE THE WARNING SIGNS TO WATCH FOR: *high fever, rashes, abdominal pain*

NOTES:

Chemotherapy Appointment – Round # ___

NOTES:

Ronnie's
Words of Wisdom

Many twists and turns in the
journey. Strap in tight, the ride will
be long and bumpy, but you are
protected by the love of God.

Chemotherapy Appointment – Round # ___

ONCOLOGIST'S NAME: DATE:

                                            TIME IN:

MEDICAL STAFF NAME: TIME OUT:

                                            TOTAL:

VITAL STATS

BP: TEMP: HT: WT: O_2 LEVEL:

PURPOSE/OBJECTIVE(S) OF APPOINTMENT:

QUESTIONS FOR MEDICAL STAFF

CHEMO DRUGS GIVEN AND TIME

DRUG: TIME START: TIME END:

   REACTION(S):

DRUG: TIME START: TIME END:

   REACTION(S):

DRUG: TIME START: TIME END:

   REACTION(S):

Chemotherapy Appointment – Round # ___

INJECTIONS GIVEN:

RIGHT BODY PART:

LEFT BODY PART:

ADDITIONAL DRUGS TO BE TAKEN FOR NAUSEA/VOMITING:

WHAT ARE THE WARNING SIGNS TO WATCH FOR: *high fever, rashes, abdominal pain*

NOTES:

Chemotherapy Appointment – Round # ___

NOTES:

Section Eleven

Radiology II
Appointment Sheet

(Post-surgery—Ultrasound and Mammogram)

Ronnie's
Words of Wisdom

This is a repeat drill—you have come this far by faith—stay strong and lean into these last few episodes of your journey—you have been moving forward! Keep up the pace... the end is near! My prayers are for positive results for you!

Radiology II Appointment – Ultrasound and Mammogram

RADIOLOGIST'S NAME:

MEDICAL STAFF NAMES:

DATE:

TIME IN:

TIME OUT:

TOTAL:

VITAL STATS

BP: TEMP: HT: WT: O_2 LEVEL:

PURPOSE/OBJECTIVE(S) OF APPOINTMENT:

QUESTIONS FOR RADIOLOGIST

NOTES:

NEXT APPOINTMENT DATE:

CONSULTATIONS NEEDED BEFORE NEXT APPOINTMENT:

Section Twelve

Radiology IIA
Appointment Sheet

(Post-surgery—MRI and CT)

Ronnie's
Words of Wisdom

Find solace in the fact that you
have been here, done it and this is
now the sequel—you shined in your
debut; now you will sparkle—
you are winning! Go, Go, Go!!!

Radiology IIA Appointment – MRI and CT

RADIOLOGIST'S NAME:

MEDICAL STAFF NAMES:

DATE:

TIME IN:

TIME OUT:

TOTAL:

VITAL STATS

BP: TEMP: HT: WT: O_2 LEVEL:

PURPOSE/OBJECTIVE(S) OF APPOINTMENT:

QUESTIONS FOR RADIOLOGIST

NOTES:

NEXT APPOINTMENT DATE:

CONSULTATIONS NEEDED BEFORE NEXT APPOINTMENT:

Section Thirteen

Radiation I
Appointment Sheet

Measuring

Radiation 1 Appointment – Measuring

TECHNICIAN'S NAME:

MEDICAL STAFF NAMES:

DATE:

TIME IN:

TIME OUT:

TOTAL:

VITAL STATS

BP: TEMP: HT: WT: O_2 LEVEL:

PURPOSE/OBJECTIVE(S) OF APPOINTMENT:

QUESTIONS FOR TECHNICIAN

TATTOO LOCATIONS:

INFORMATION TO RECEIVE:

EXPLANATION OF PROCEDURE:

Radiation I Appointment – Measuring

MEASUREMENTS:

EFFECTS OF RADIATION:

PRE-RADIATION INSTRUCTIONS:

WHAT TO WEAR:

NOTES:

Radiation 1 Appointment – Measuring

NOTES:

NEXT APPOINTMENT DATE:

CONSULTATIONS NEEDED BEFORE NEXT APPOINTMENT:

Section Fourteen

Radiation II
Appointment Sheets

Rounds

Ronnie's
Words of Wisdom

Your radiation appointments are times to breathe; take in your surroundings; be grateful. Relax for a moment during your treatment.

Radiation II Appointment – Round # ___

TECHNICIAN'S NAME:

MEDICAL STAFF NAMES:

DATE:

TIME IN:

TIME OUT:

TOTAL:

VITAL STATS

BP: TEMP: HT: WT: O_2 LEVEL:

PURPOSE/OBJECTIVE(S) OF APPOINTMENT:

QUESTIONS FOR TECHNICIAN

NOTES:

NEXT APPOINTMENT DATE:

CONSULTATIONS NEEDED BEFORE NEXT APPOINTMENT:

You have been grinding along;
time to slow down a bit
and get re-centered.

Radiation II Appointment – Round # ___

TECHNICIAN'S NAME: ___

MEDICAL STAFF NAMES: ___

DATE: ___
TIME IN: ___
TIME OUT: ___
TOTAL: ___

VITAL STATS

BP: TEMP: HT: WT: O_2 LEVEL:

PURPOSE/OBJECTIVE(S) OF APPOINTMENT:

QUESTIONS FOR TECHNICIAN

NOTES:

NEXT APPOINTMENT DATE:

CONSULTATIONS NEEDED BEFORE NEXT APPOINTMENT:

Ronnie's Words of Wisdom

You will have many appointments—they will be quick. Take a moment and be grateful.

Radiation II Appointment – Round # ___

TECHNICIAN'S NAME:

DATE:

TIME IN:

MEDICAL STAFF NAMES:

TIME OUT:

TOTAL:

VITAL STATS

BP: TEMP: HT: WT: O_2 LEVEL:

PURPOSE/OBJECTIVE(S) OF APPOINTMENT:

QUESTIONS FOR TECHNICIAN

NOTES:

NEXT APPOINTMENT DATE:

CONSULTATIONS NEEDED BEFORE NEXT APPOINTMENT:

Radiation II Appointment – Round # ___

TECHNICIAN'S NAME: _____

DATE: _____

TIME IN: _____

MEDICAL STAFF NAMES: _____

TIME OUT: _____

TOTAL: _____

VITAL STATS

BP: TEMP: HT: WT: O_2 LEVEL:

PURPOSE/OBJECTIVE(S) OF APPOINTMENT:

QUESTIONS FOR TECHNICIAN

NOTES:

NEXT APPOINTMENT DATE:

CONSULTATIONS NEEDED BEFORE NEXT APPOINTMENT:

Ronnie's
Words of Wisdom

You know what to expect now.
Have peace with understanding
that you will have your
healthy body back soon.

Radiation II Appointment – Round # ___

TECHNICIAN'S NAME: DATE:

TIME IN:

MEDICAL STAFF NAMES: TIME OUT:

TOTAL:

VITAL STATS

BP: TEMP: HT: WT: O_2 LEVEL:

PURPOSE/OBJECTIVE(S) OF APPOINTMENT:

QUESTIONS FOR TECHNICIAN

NOTES:

NEXT APPOINTMENT DATE:

CONSULTATIONS NEEDED BEFORE NEXT APPOINTMENT:

Not sure where you are in
your treatments, but I do know
that you are awesome, and
you are persevering!
Keep up the good work.

Radiation II Appointment – Round # ____

TECHNICIAN'S NAME:

DATE:

TIME IN:

MEDICAL STAFF NAMES:

TIME OUT:

TOTAL:

VITAL STATS

BP: TEMP: HT: WT: O_2 LEVEL:

PURPOSE/OBJECTIVE(S) OF APPOINTMENT:

QUESTIONS FOR TECHNICIAN

NOTES:

NEXT APPOINTMENT DATE:

CONSULTATIONS NEEDED BEFORE NEXT APPOINTMENT:

Ronnie's
Words of Wisdom

Take time during this treatment
to jot down five things you are
thankful for—I am thankful for
you hanging in there!

Radiation II Appointment – Round # ___

TECHNICIAN'S NAME:

DATE:

TIME IN:

MEDICAL STAFF NAMES:

TIME OUT:

TOTAL:

VITAL STATS

BP: TEMP: HT: WT: O_2 LEVEL:

PURPOSE/OBJECTIVE(S) OF APPOINTMENT:

QUESTIONS FOR TECHNICIAN

NOTES:

NEXT APPOINTMENT DATE:

CONSULTATIONS NEEDED BEFORE NEXT APPOINTMENT:

Ronnie's Words of Wisdom

Do you have a mantra to quell your mind? Think of a short phrase you can repeat to keep yourself centered. Mine was: "I believe, I believe, I believe."

Radiation II Appointment – Round # ___

TECHNICIAN'S NAME: _____   DATE: _____

MEDICAL STAFF NAMES: _____   TIME IN: _____

_____   TIME OUT: _____

                                               TOTAL: _____

VITAL STATS

BP: _____   TEMP: _____   HT: _____   WT: _____ O_2 LEVEL: _____

PURPOSE/OBJECTIVE(S) OF APPOINTMENT:

_____

_____

_____

_____

_____

QUESTIONS FOR TECHNICIAN

_____

_____

_____

_____

NOTES:

_____

_____

_____

_____

NEXT APPOINTMENT DATE: _____

CONSULTATIONS NEEDED BEFORE NEXT APPOINTMENT:

_____

Radiation II Appointment – Round # ___

TECHNICIAN'S NAME:

MEDICAL STAFF NAMES:

DATE:

TIME IN:

TIME OUT:

TOTAL:

VITAL STATS

BP: TEMP: HT: WT: O_2 LEVEL:

PURPOSE/OBJECTIVE(S) OF APPOINTMENT:

QUESTIONS FOR TECHNICIAN

NOTES:

NEXT APPOINTMENT DATE:

CONSULTATIONS NEEDED BEFORE NEXT APPOINTMENT:

Ronnie's Words of Wisdom

If you are completing your
radiation treatments, be grateful
and give thanks to the medical team
for providing excellent care.
Give yourself a pat on the back—
well done!!

Radiation II Appointment – Round # ___

TECHNICIAN'S NAME:

DATE:

TIME IN:

MEDICAL STAFF NAMES:

TIME OUT:

TOTAL:

VITAL STATS

BP: TEMP: HT: WT: O_2 LEVEL:

PURPOSE/OBJECTIVE(S) OF APPOINTMENT:

QUESTIONS FOR TECHNICIAN

NOTES:

NEXT APPOINTMENT DATE:

CONSULTATIONS NEEDED BEFORE NEXT APPOINTMENT:

Section Fifteen

Medical History Sheets

Medications, Allergies, and Surgeries

Medical History – Medications, Allergies, and Surgeries

MEDICATION LIST—DATE

MEDICATION ALLERGIES

OTHER ALLERGIES

Medical History – Medications, Allergies, and Surgeries

SURGICAL HISTORY—DATE

SURGERY:

DR:
DATE:

SURGERY:

DR:
DATE:

SURGERY:

DR:
DATE:

SURGERY:

DR:
DATE:

SURGERY:

DR:
DATE:

SURGERY:

DR:
DATE:

SURGERY:

DR:
DATE:

SURGERY:

DR:
DATE:

SURGERY:

DR:
DATE:

SURGERY:

DR:
DATE:

SURGERY:

DR:
DATE:

SURGERY:

DR:
DATE:

Section Sixteen

Contact Sheets

Physicians, Family, Friends

Contacts – Physicians, Family, Friends

PHYSICIANS

NAME:

PHONE:

EMAIL:

ADDRESS:

NAME:

PHONE:

EMAIL:

ADDRESS:

NAME:

PHONE:

EMAIL:

ADDRESS:

NAME:

PHONE:

EMAIL:

ADDRESS:

NAME:

PHONE:

EMAIL:

ADDRESS:

NAME:

PHONE:

EMAIL:

ADDRESS:

NAME:

PHONE:

EMAIL:

ADDRESS:

NAME:

PHONE:

EMAIL:

ADDRESS:

PHARMACY

NAME:

PHONE:

EMAIL:

ADDRESS:

PHARMACY

NAME:

PHONE:

EMAIL:

ADDRESS:

Contacts – Physicians, Family, Friends

FAMILY AND FRIENDS

NAME:

PHONE:

EMAIL:

ADDRESS:

NAME:

PHONE:

EMAIL:

ADDRESS:

NAME:

PHONE:

EMAIL:

ADDRESS:

NAME:

PHONE:

EMAIL:

ADDRESS:

NAME:

PHONE:

EMAIL:

ADDRESS:

NAME:

PHONE:

EMAIL:

ADDRESS:

NAME:

PHONE:

EMAIL:

ADDRESS:

NAME:

PHONE:

EMAIL:

ADDRESS:

NAME:

PHONE:

EMAIL:

ADDRESS:

NAME:

PHONE:

EMAIL:

ADDRESS:

Acknowledgements

My Appointment Notebook was born out of necessity. I found it necessary to have all my medical information in one place during my cancer journey so that I could keep track of the information. This made my cancer journey less cumbersome. As I thought about how to organize the pages and set up the format, I bounced the idea off of a couple of My Tribe members. I am indebted for their insights and suggestions to make *My Appointment Notebook* a reality.

Angie Martin, you were my creative genius who never tired of my "What if's…" or my "How can I…." Your feedback about my ideas was always sincere, functional and insightful. You always helped me view the project from different perspectives and this in turn yielded the final completed product. Many thanks for your guided suggestions.

Angela Lott Bower, you were my medical resource who made sure that all areas from the medical aspect were covered. Your keen sense of the medical field helped me to make sure that I left no stone unturned. I was grateful for your thoroughness and your ability to help me keep *My Appointment Notebook* practical and functional. Your feedback was greatly appreciated.

I have to acknowledge my dynamic team at Franklin Green Publishing, Scott Spiewak, Heidi Jensen and Kent Jensen. You all helped me to hone *My Appointment Notebook* into the product that it came to be. Your attention to detail and organization made my edits flow smoothly. Your creative style for the layout was fitting for me and my product. I am thankful that I had such a cohesive team working in my favor.

We now know that all things
are possible if we believe that God
has a plan. All that we have to do
is trust and believe in Him!

Words of Gratitude

Hello Again,

I wanted to share a few words of gratitude with you for staying strong, hanging in there and most importantly moving forward. You did a thing—you kept going, taking notes, asking questions, and following directions. Now you are on the other side with a new attitude and outlook about this thing we call life. You are a winner and a survivor—Celebrate!

It is always some kind of trauma that causes us to stop and pause. And pause you did for a split second to take it all in; and then kept it moving forward. I am so proud of your perseverance and tenacity in your journey—what a feat! Well done!

Be grateful for your support team however that may be comprised. They were integral in your ability to keep pushing to make it through—nothing like a great support team no matter what you call them! I am sending my love to them—as well as to you.

Just something to think about: you were diagnosed with breast cancer, and you demonstrated resilience beyond measure. I am so happy and proud of you for just moving through the process. Do not ever think that something is impossible. We now know that all things are possible if we believe that God has a plan. All that we have to do is trust and believe in Him!

My prayer for you is for continued good health and happiness. Try to motivate someone else who may not have the same drive as you. And that good measure will be returned to you tenfold—or maybe, it already has!

Be well and keep moving—

Love ya!

V. Ronnie Laughlin

www.ronnielaughlin.com

Ronnie's Words of Wisdom

You thrived and survived
this journey. Live your new
healthy life with the same vigor
you used to navigate your journey!
You did it! Congrats!

Glossary of Terms

Adjuvant Therapy: A primary type of treatment that involves surgery first for the excision of the tumor, then radiation as prophylaxis (prevention).

Anesthesia (propofol): A drug used to induce sleep during surgery.

Angiogram: A way to view blood vessels for guidance during various procedures.

Benign: Non-cancerous.

BIRADS: Breast Imaging Reporting Data System. A system that categorizes breast images. The categories range from 0 (findings are unclear; more images are needed) to 6 (cancer was diagnosed using a biopsy).

BRCA: Breast Cancer gene test. It is used to determine the presence of BRCA 1 or BRCA 2 gene.

BRCA 1 Gene: Linked to triple negative breast cancer—a very aggressive and deadly form of breast cancer that can increase the risk of ovarian, pancreatic, gallbladder, bile duct and melanoma cancers. Usually inherited.

BRCA 2 Gene: Associated with cancer that are generally estrogen receptor positive.

Cancer-Related Fatigue (CRF): Extreme and long-lasting fatigue associated with chemotherapy. It is unlike fatigue from being tired; sleep does not help CRF.

CBC (complete blood count): Blood analysis done to determine blood cell count. CBC is monitored during chemo to ensure adequate white blood cell count.

Clip/Marker: A marker placed subcutaneously (under the skin) that helps the surgeon more easily find the site when surgery is warranted for breast cancer.

Contrast: Liquid material injected into the vein via an IV (intravenous) to help highlight any abnormal areas of breast tissue or any other abnormal tissue during an MRI (magnetic resonance image) or CT scan. The ingredient in the contrast is called gadolinium.

Core Needle Biopsy: A hollow needle that is used to remove pieces of breast tissue.

CT (computerized tomography) Scan: A scan typically done to diagnose tumors, investigate internal bleeding, or check for internal injuries or damage. The scan combines a series of x-ray images from different angles around the body. Computer processing is used to create cross sectional images or slices of the tissue they are focusing on. The CT scan gives more detailed information than a plain X-ray. The CT scan is considered an asset to the cancer profession for its detailed imaging.

Dexamethasone: Drug used during chemotherapy to help quell nausea and vomiting. It can also be used for other medical ailments such as allergies, asthma, and skin diseases.

Echocardiogram (ECHO): A graphic outline of the movement of the heart's valves and chambers through the use of a hand-held wand guided over the chest assessing the heart's anatomy and function.

Fibroadenoma: A solid, not fluid filled tumor caused by a deviation or change during normal development of breast tissue. The breast lobules become hyperplastic (over plastic). This change can be related to estrogen, progesterone, pregnancy and lactation.

Filgrastim: A drug that stimulates bone marrow to make new white blood cells that are measured via the white blood count (WBC).

Gait: Your walking strides.

Heparin: An anticoagulant (prevents blood clotting). It is used in the port-a-catheter to keep it open or patent between chemo treatments.

HER: Human Epidermal growth factor Receptor (a protein).

HER 2: Protein that promotes the growth of cancer cells.

Immunohistochemistry (IHC): A test used to determine cell type and organ of origin. The test can be performed on breast tissue samples that are suspected of being malignant (cancerous). The sample may be tested for HER2 receptors and/or hormone receptors.

In situ: Original place.

Intraductal Carcinoma: Aka, ductal carcinoma in situ (DCIS); cancer in its original place; it has not spread.

Intravenous: In the vein.

Keloids: Thick raised scar on skin.

Lesion: A tumor.

Mammogram: A visual representation of the breasts using various views to discern the structure/landscape of the breast and determine the tissue, density, identify masses and locate malignant and benign masses in the breast. Low-energy X-rays are used to examine the breast for diagnosis or screening or the location of a marker for future surgery.

Margins: Typical, a rim of tissue around the site anywhere from 1-2 millimeters in circumference.

Metastasized: Spread.

Methylene Blue Dye: A dye injected into sentinel nodes which has radioactive properties to detect cancer. The dye can be seen in urine after being flushed from body.

Methylphenidate: An FDA-approved drug for ADHD in children and adults. It is also a psychostimulant drug used to treat fatigue in patients with cancer, for which there is no gold standard.

Mucositis: The inflammation of the mucosal (mouth) region.

Neoadjuvant Therapy: A type of chemotherapy approach that is used ahead of surgery to help shrink a cancerous tumor or even kill cancerous tissue that is not visible on imaging tests. When neoadjuvant therapy is used, doctors may also be looking at how the tumor responds to the drugs, and this can guide the treatment.

Neutropenia: Low white blood cell count.

Nystagmus: Rapid side-to-side uncontrolled eye movements.

Olanzapine: A drug used in chemotherapy treatment to quell nausea and vomiting.

Osteopenia: Brittle bones.

Palpate: To touch.

Patent: To keep open.

Pathogens: Germs.

Port-a-Catheter: A device that is inserted under the skin opposite the cancerous site that delivers chemotherapy drugs without harming veins in the patient. It is connected to the large vein that leads to the heart for distribution of the drugs throughout the body.

Positive Prognostic Indicators: Factors that contribute to good outcomes after treatment, e.g., healthy status, good diet, no history of illnesses.

Positive/Complete Clinical Response (P/CCR): Evidence that a tumor/lesion has been resolved (dissolved) after chemotherapy. The cancer is no longer detectable at the site.

Prophylactic: Just in case/preventative.

Prophylaxis: Prevention.

Sentinel Node: The first node located under the arm pit that a tumor will spread to. It is tested to determine if cancer is in other nodes in the lymph system.

Sonogram: Use of sound waves to see structures/organs.

Subcutaneous: Under the skin; a pocket made under the skin to insert a device.

Tumor Board: A group of hospital professionals consisting of Pathologists, Surgeons, Medical and Radiation Oncologists, Plastic Surgeons, Urologists, Gynecologists, Genetic counselor; and anyone else specific for the type of cancer of the patient in various areas of Oncology and Medicine. They typically meet weekly to discuss all cancer cases at a hospital and to determine the best possible cancer treatment and care plan for an individual patient, based on the most current research and best evidence-based practices.

Wire Localization: Use of a fine wire to mark the site of a tumor. It can guide the surgeon to ensure that they have the correct spot to remove the tissue or for the biopsy.

Ronnie's
Words of Wisdom

Positivity got you through your journey. Be sure to project positivity daily in all that you do! Staying positive is imperative!

Notes

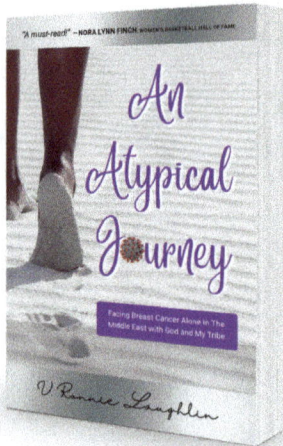

"A must-read!" —NORA LYNN FINCH WOMEN'S BASKETBALL HALL OF FAME

An Atypical Journey

Facing Breast Cancer Alone in The Middle East with God and My Tribe

V Ronnie Laughlin

Order Here

VRL
RonnieLaughlin.com

An Atypical Journey - Facing Breast Cancer Alone in The Middle East with God and My Tribe
V. Ronnie Laughlin, SLP

At the height of the COVID-19 pandemic, Ronnie was diagnosed with breast cancer while working in the Middle East. Ronnie had no other option but to drive herself to chemo treatments as the pandemic shut down the world. As a former Division I basketball player and now a Speech Pathologist, Ronnie gathered everything she learned on and off the court - sheer determination, life trials and victories, her medical knowledge, and her dynamic faith. Ronnie recalled the lessons her parents and former coach, Coach Kay Yow, taught throughout this season in her life—they were a gift. Ronnie had a Tribe of friends who motivated and encouraged her along the way, as she knew this journey would be anything but typical. Collectively, Ronnie used every experience to write this outstanding inspirational book on how she faced her breast cancer challenge "alone" during a worldwide pandemic. Ronnie wants you to know that you are never alone in your journey—you always have someone by your side. This book is full of remarkable insight, analysis, and suggestions such as staying grateful, staying positive, staying mobile via exercise, eating healthy, and keeping track of all your appointments when you are exhausted. This book illuminates the unknown, eases one's anxiety, and negates the many surprises and fears that cancer brings. An Atypical Journey is an inspirational book for patients and their families facing one of life's most challenging journeys - cancer.

Ronnie Speaks On:

- Breast Cancer Awareness
- Resilience Through Great Trials
- Power of Support; Tribe from Afar
- Driving to Chemo Treatments Alone
- Importance of Fitness and Healthy Eating
- Game Plan—Healthy Thought Process
- Team Managment and Communication
- Insightful Tips That Bring Relief

Ronnie Laughlin is a gifted athlete, who excelled in sports—basketball, volleyball, and track and field. A former Division I Basketball player she played for Peace College and North Carolina State University. Ronnie graduated from NCSU with an undergraduate degree in Speech Communication. Ronnie obtained her Master of Arts Degree from Louisiana State University. Ronnie has worked in various settings including schools, universities, hospitals and clinics. Ronnie has been a color analyst for radio and television broadcasts. She is now a Speech Pathologist working in the Middle East helping children, adolescents, and adults to communicate effectively. Despite being diagnosed with breast cancer during the height of the COVID-19 pandemic Ronnie wanted to write this book to share with others how she coped with her diagnosis. Ronnie is an avid golfer and a Leaderboard member for Women of Color Golf (WOCG) in Tampa, Florida.

To win against cancer, or any imposing obstacle, one must engage physically, mentally, emotionally, and spiritually. Ronnie's game plan includes action plans in all four realms. She researched online, communicated with close friends, drank gallons of water, ate high protein foods, exercised, and talked with God. Philippians 4:11-13 became Ronnie's mantra-Lord, may your will be done. There is undeniable comfort in knowing that whatever happens to us is part of God's plan if we are following His will by putting Him first, giving Him the credit, claiming His faithfulness, thanking Him for all things because we trust that He will work everything according to His will (Romans 8:28). God's plan for Ronnie is revealed throughout **An Atypical Journey**. *It's a must read for you or your loved one going through cancer!*

-Nora Lynn Finch
Women's Basketball Hall of Fame

For More Information Contact Ronnie at info@ronnielaughlin.com

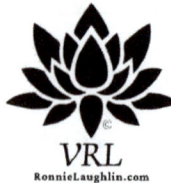

"When Life Kicks You, Let It Kick You Forward!"
-Kay Yow

10% of Proceeds Goes to
Kay Yow Cancer Fund.

Kay Yow Cancer Fund

4804 Page Creek Lane, Suite 118

Durham, NC 27703

Website: kayyow.com

Jenny Palmateer, CEO

"Your Attitude Determines Your Altitude."
-Kay Yow